HAIR LOSS

EXPLAINED AND ANALYSED

(The Homoeopathic Way)

HAIR LOSS
EXPLAINED AND ANALYSED
(The Homoeopathic Way)

PROF. DR. FAROKH J. MASTER
L.C.E.H(Bom) Gold medalist, F.H.M.A. (U.K.)
Prof. of Medicine Bombay University

Consulting Physician:
Bombay Hospital, K.E.M. Hospital,
B.D. Petit Parsee Gen.Hospital,
Tata Service, Indian Navy, O.N.G.C.

B. Jain Publishers (P) Ltd.
USE — EUROPE — INDIA

HAIR LOSS EXPLAINED AND ANALYSED

First Edition: 1992
13th Impression: 2016

Published by Kuldeep Jain for
B. JAIN PUBLISHERS (P) LTD.
B. Jain House, D-157, Sector-63,
NOIDA-201307, U.P. (INDIA)
Tel.: +91-120-4933333 • Email: info@bjain.com
Website: www.bjain.com

Printed in India
B B Press Noida
ISBN: 978-81-319-0245-5

DEDICATION

This book is dedicated to my friend "Mr. **Satish Arora**"

Just like four leaved Clovers

Are hard to find,

There seldom is

One of your kind.

PREFACE

Five years ago when I announced my textbook on skin diseases, I had decided that I should publish a separate booklet on hair loss as this complaint is one of the most commonest complaints presented to any physician in the metropolis.

The market is flooded these days with many wonder drugs. Hairoils Shampoos, lotions, the arrival of which is announced with much publicity and very soon the people come to know the futility of such a gimmick.

The thing which has withstood since last one hundred and eighty years against all odds is the science of constitutional Homoeopethic Medicine. In this booklet I have described the anatomy, physiological functions, various diseases of the hair. Homoeopathic therapeutics from various materia medica's Repertory of Hair loss from various Repertories and Clinical cases.

I hope this will be accepted by the profession like my previous publications.

DR. FAROKH JAMSHED MASTER

11-9-91

VATCHA GANDHY MEMORIAL BLDG No. 1

HUGHES RD.

BOMBAY-400007

ACKNOWLEDGEMENT

My sincere thanks to:

1. Kuldeep Jain
2. Premchand Jain
3. Ashok Jain

who have always encouraged me in my efforts to write a book.

Dr. Kripal Singh Bakshi and his dynamic Son Dr. Sunny Bakshi for their constant guidance.

My Clinical assistants:

Dr. Niloufer Bamji
Dr. Kamal Kodia
Dr. Afshan Deshmukh
Dr. Vincent Castelino
Dr. Nilufer Panthaky
Dr. Shailen Petigara
Dr. Kamal Rustomjee

Dr. Shahrukh Pavri
Dr. Sharmila Lulla
Dr. Diana Minbattiwalla
DR. Zubin Marolia
Dr. Devika Pooran
Dr. Swati Kanakiya

Miss. Roda Bandrawalla for typing the manuscript.

Mr. Noshir Dadrewalla who is omnipotent in all my endevours.

CONTENTS

CONTENTS

1

DISEASES OF THE SKIN APPENDAGES

DISEASES OF THE HAIR

Normal human hairs can be classified according to cyclical phases of growth. Anagen hairs are growing hairs, catagent hairs are those undergoing transition from the growing to the resting stage, and telogen hairs are resting hairs, which remain in the follicles for variable lengths of time before they fall out.

Anagen hairs grow for some three years (1000 days - Orentreich), with the limits generally set between two and six years. The follicular cells grow, divide, and become keratinized to form growing hairs. The base of the hair shaft is soft and moist. A darkly pigmented portion is evident just above the hair builb.

Catagen hairs are in a transitional phase, lasting a week or two, in which all growth activity ceases, with formation of the "club" hair.

Telogen hairs, also known as club hairs, are resting hairs, which continue in this state some three to four months (100 days - Orentreich) before they are pushed out of the hair follicle by the hairs growing underneath them, or pulled out by a hair brush or other mechanical means.

Among human hairs plucked from normal scalp, 90 per cent are anagen hairs and 10 per cent catagen or telogen hairs. It has been estimated that the scalp normally contains 100,000 hairs, therefore the average number of hairs shed daily is 100. Contrary to popular belief, neither shaving nor menstruation has any effect upon hair growth rate.

Human hair is also designated as lanugo, vellus, or terminal hair. Lanugo hair is the fine hair present on the body of the

11

fetus. This is replaced by the vellus and terminal hairs. Vellus hairs are fine (fuzz), usually light-colored, and characteristically seen on children's faces and arms. Terminal hairs are coarse, thick, and dark, except in blonds. Hair occurs on all skin surfaces except the palms, soles, glans, and prepuce. Terminal hairs are always present on men's face, chest, and abdomen, but vellus hairs usually predominate on these sites in women.

ALOPECIA

ALOPECIA AREATA

CLINICAL FEATURES. Alopecia areata (in French, pelade) is characterized by rapid and complete loss of hair in one, or more often several, round or oval patches, usually on the scalp, the bearded area, the eyebrows, the eyelashes, and rarely on other hairy areas of the body. Commonly the patches are from 1 to 5 cm in diameter. A few resting hairs may be found within the patches, and the surface may be slightly depressed. Early in the course there may be sparing of grey hair. Nearly always the hair loss is patchy in distribution; however, cases may present in a diffuse pattern. At the periphery of the bald patch are loose hairs that may be broken off near the scalp, leaving short stumps. When they are pulled out a tapered, attenuated bulb is seen as a result of atrophy of that portion: hence the term "exclamation point" hair. These telogen hairs are usually located at the periphery of the bald patch. However, the problem arises in the anagen phase when damage to the hair shaft induces early catagen and telogen phases. The tendency is for spontaneous recovery in patients whose age at onset was after puberty. At first the regrowing hairs are downy and light in color; later they are replaced by stronger and darker hair with full growth. In some patients there is progression of the disease, with the development of new bald patches, until there is a total loss of scalp hair (alopecia totalis). When hair has been lost over the entire body, including the scalp, the designation is alopecia universalis. Alopecia areata usually occurs without associated disease. However, there is a higher incidence than usual in patients with atopic dermatitis, Down's syndrome, and such autoimmune diseases as thyroiditis and vitiligo.

12

ETIOLOGY. Although Celsus described and named alopecia areata some 20 centuries ago, its cause is still unknown. Most evidence points toward its being an autoimmune disease modified by genetic factos and aggravated by emotional stress.

Many studies have documented abnormal cellumediated immune factors in alopecia areata. There is an increased suppressor T-cell function in patients experiencing regrowth. In the inflammatory perifollicular infiltrate seen in active cases, helper cells predominate. Stress has been regarded for years as a possible initiator, and if it does play a role, it may be as an instigator of an immune mechanism.

Genetic susceptibility appears to be a factor, as suggested by a possible HLA association. Nearly 25 per cent of patients have a positive family history; there are reports of twins with alopecia areata; and certain populations may be at higher risk. Hordinsky et al reported a white American family in which three members from two generations had alopecia, areata in one and universalis in two.

Alopecia areata has been associated with several autoimmune diseases, including chronic lymphocytic thyroiditis (Hashimoto's disease), pernicious anemia, Addison's disease, vitiligo, and several of the connective tissue diseases. The presence of antibodies against thyroglobulin, parietal cells, adrenal cells, and thyroid cells has been demonstrated.

TELOGEN EFFLUVIUM

Kligman has defined telogen effluvium as the early and excessive loss of normal club hairs from resting follicles in the scalp. This excessive hair loss results from the traumatization of the normal hair by some stimulus (e.g., surgery, parturition, fever, drugs, traction) which precipitates the anagen phase into catagen and telogen phases in short order. Kligman points out that during this process the follicle itself is not diseased, and inflammation is absent.

Whatever the cause, telogen effluvium usually has a latent period of from two to four months; the hair loss is noted by the

13

patient as "lots of hairs coming out by the roots." Loss is diffuse and only infrequently caused noticeable thinning of the hair, since it only rarely involves more than 50 per cent of the hairs. Increased hair loss is noted by the patient before signs of alopecia. The normal telogen count may vary from 5 to 20 per cent; the diagnosis of telogen effluvium is usually justified only if the telogen count is over 25 per cent.

The normal average daily loss is influenced by such factors as age, sex, race, and probably other genetic factors. The total number of hairs on scalp is estimated to be about 100,000; of these, aproximately 100 hairs are lost daily. In telogen effluvium estimates of loss vary from 120 to over 400.

In telogen effluvium the majority of the follicles continue in the anagen phase. The club hair is shed because the new hair generated in the anagen phase is pushing out the old club hair.

There is no specific therapy for telogen effluvium; it will stop spontaneously within a few weeks and the hair will regrow. If it threatens to become cosmetically significant, it can be arrested promptly in the majority of cases by constitutional homoeopathic treatment. Regrowth begins within a week or so. The prognosis is good if a specific event can be pinpointed as a probable cause.

Traction telogen **effluvium** was emphasized by Steck; it results chiefly from tight braiding, or winding hair too tightly on curlers or otherwise.

Postpartum telogen effluvium has been found to begin between two and five months postpartum. Often the hair loss is first noted over the anterior third of the scalp, although loss is in a diffuse pattern. The hair loss continues for some two to six months or longer. A complete regrowth eventually occurs.

Postnatal telogen effluvium of infants may occur between birth and the first four months of age. Usually regrowth occurs by six months of age.

Psychogenic telogen effluvium has been found by Kligman to differ from ordinary telogen effluvium; it persists longer, and there may be repeated episodes of lessening loss. The sudden loss of all the scalp hair after shock is believed to be of alopecia areata type.

Postfebrile telogen effluvium is familiar after febrile illnesses such pneumonia. Here again hair loss begins some two to four months after the febrile episode. Telogen counts may be well over 50 per cent. Regrowth is the course.

Drug-induced telogen effluvium has been noted with heparin, coumarin, triparanol, thioureas, carbamazepine, lithium carbonate,, indo-methacin, allopurinol, gentamicin, metoprolol, isotretinioin, etretinate, levodopa, and propranolol.

Other causes of telogen effluvium have been noted. The most dramatic has been kwashikor. Goette and Odom have reported telogen effluvium in people on weight reduction programs and crash diets, secondary to protein deprivation.

ANAGEN EFFLUVIUM

Kligman has observed that anagen effluvium is seen frequently following the administration of cancer chemotherapeutic agents such as the antimetabolites, alkylating agents, and mitotic inhibitors. Severe loss is frequently seen with doxorubicin, the nitrosureas, and cyclophos-phamide. When high doses are given, loss of anagen hairs occurs almost immediately or in one or two weeks. It becomes clinically most apparent in one to two months. The hair shafts are abruptly thinned at the time of maximum drug effect, and when the very thin portion reaches the surface, the hair shafts all break at about the same time. Many hairs may also, if the bulb itself is damaged, separate at the bulb itself and come out. It is to be noted that only growing ("anagen") hairs are subject to this type of change. With cessation of drug therapy the follicle resumes its normal activity within a few weeks; the process is entirely reversible. It is apparent that mitotic inhibition only stops the reproduction of matrix cells, but does not permanently destroy the hair. A pressure cuff applied around the scalp during chemotherapy can prevent such anagen arrest. In addition to the cytotoxic agents, various chemicals such as thallium and boron may induce anagen effluvium.

15

MALE PATTERN ALOPECIA

(Androgenetic Alopecia)

Male pattern alopecia or male pattern baldness (common baldness) was called androgenetic alopecia by Orentreich in 1960. It shows itself during the twenties or early thirties by gradual loss of hair, chiefly from the vertex and frontotemporal regions. At any time after puberty the process may begin subtly, and the presence of "whisker" hair at the temples may be the first sign of impending male pattern alopecia. The anterior hair line recedes on each side, in the "Geheimratswinkeln" ("professor angles"), so that the forehead becomes high. Eventually the entire top of the scalp may become devoid of hair. Several patterns of this type of hair loss occur, but the most frequent is the biparietal recession with loss of hair on the vertex. The rate of hair loss varies among individuals. A sudden hair loss may occur in the twenties and then proceed relentlessly though very slowly for a number of years. The follicles produce finer and lighter terminal hairs until a complete cessation of terminal hair growth results. Vellus hairs on the scalp, however, continue to grow and become more prominent because of the absence of terminal hairs. The parietal and occipital areas are usually spared permanently.

The exact mechanisms responsible for androgenetic alopecia are still unkown; however, there is no doubt that inherited factors and the effect of androgens on the hair are most responsible.

In addition to heredity, male-pattern alopecia is dependent upon adequte androgen stimulation at a particular age of the individual. Hamilton has shown that eunuchs do not develop baldness provided they are castrated before or during adolescence; if they are given androgen therapy, baldness may develop.

Vera Price has extensively reviewed testosterone metabolism in the skin. The 5 - reduction of testosterone is increased in the scalp of balding individuals, yielding increased dihydrotestosterone. It has been suggested that high dihydrotestosterone levels in the genetically marked hair follicles initiate baldness by inhibiting adenyl cyclase.

16

ANDROGENETIC ALOPECIA IN WOMEN

The pattern of hair loss is quite different in women. Women generally have diffuse hair loss throughout the mid-scalp, sparing the frontal hair line except for slight recession.

The cause is now believed to be a genetic predisposition in combination with an excessive androgen response, even though levels of circulating testosterone are as a rule not elevated. Rook and Ebling classify this form of alopecia with the androgen-dependent syndromes.

OTHER FORMS OF ALOPECIA

Complete or partial loss of scalp hair is found in various forms and is caused by many factors. Some forms of alopecia are herewith described briefly.

Trichotillomania is a neurotic practice of plucking or breaking hair from scalp or eyelashes. This is seen in mostly girls under 10, but boys, and adults of either sex, may it too.

Hot comb alopecia is seen in black women who straighten their hair with hot combs for cosmetic purposes. Lo Presti and his associates state that the alopecia develops characteristically on the crown and spreads peripherally to form a large oval area of partial hair loss. The hot petrolatum used with the iron causes thermal damage to the hair follice, leading ultimately to destruction of the entire follicle and a follicular scar. In time significant hair loss occurs if this type of hair straightening is continued.

Traction alopecia is probably of the same mechanism as that of telogen effluvium, but is limited to areas thus traumatized. It occurs from prolonged tension on the hair either from wearing the hair tightly braided or in a ponytail, pulling the hair to straighten it, rolling curlers too tightly, or form the habit of twisting the hairs with the fingers.

Pressure alopecia occurs frequently on the occipital areas in babies lying on their backs. In adults, it is seen most often after prolonged pressure on the scalp during general anesthesia, with

17

the head fixed in one position. It may also occur in chronically ill persons after prolonged bed rest in one position, which causes persistent pressure upon one part of the scalp.

Loose anagen syndrome, described by Price in 1989, is a disorder in which anagen hairs may be pulled from the scalp with little effort. Price reported that it occurs mostly in blond girls. It improves with age.

Alopecia syphilitica has a typical motheaten appearance on the occipital scalp. Other areas such as the eyebrows and eyelashes and body hair may be involved. The alopecia may be the first sign of a syphilis infection. Its distinct appearance is specific.

Follicular mucinosis (alopecia mucinosa) most commonly occurs on the scalp or bread area and manifests as deposition of mucin in the outer root sheath and sebaceous glands. The inflammatory re-action produces alopecia, and at times hypopigmentation.

The primary cases (i.e., unassociated with underlying disease) occur either as a localized lesions of the head or neck that usually resolve within a year, or as more generalized lesions with a longer course. Young people are primarily affected.

A secondary type exists, in which there is associated lymphoma, most often mycosis fungoides. Usually, in these cases, lesions are widespread and chronic, and occur in older patients.

Inflammatory alopecia may be seen in lichen simplex chronicus and various eczematous changes on the scalp, including kerion. Discoid lupus erythematosus, lichen planopilaris, sarcodosis, and folliculitis decalvans are the commonest inflammatory causes of cicatricial alopecia.

Vascular or neurologic alopecia, most often of the lower extremities, may be seen in diabetes mellitus or atherosclerosis. In meralgia paresthetica there may be alopecia of the anesthetic area of the outer thigh.

18

Tinea capitis is usually manifested by one or several patches of alopecia with scaling, erythema, or pustulation. The hairs are broken off just above the scalp.

Endocrinologic alopecia may occur in various endocrinologic disorders. In hypothyroidism the hair becomes coarse, dry brittle, and sparse. Freinkel and Freinkel found in six such cases that the proportion of telogen hairs was three to seven times higher than the normal 10 per cent. In hyperthyrodism the hair becomes extremely fine and sparse. Oral contraceptives have been implicated in some instances of androgenetic alopecia. It develops in predisposed women who are usually taking androgeneic progestogens. It is advisable to discontinue the androgen-dominant pill and substitute an estrogen-dominant oral contraceptive. Some women develop telogen effluvium two to four months after discontinuing anovulatory agents, which is analogous to postpartum alopecia.

Tumour alopecia refers to hair loss in the immediate vicinity of either benign or malignant tumors of the scalp. Syringomas, nerve sheath myxomas, and steatocystoma multiplex are benign tumors that may be limited to the scalp and cause alopecia.

Alopecia neoplastica is the designation given to hair loss from metastatic tumors, most often from breast carcinoma.

Menopausal alopecia is held to be identical with male-pattern (androgenic) baldness by Maguire and Kligment.

Drug alopecia resulting from use of thallium, colchicine, and various antineoplastic cytotoxic agents such as vinblastine, chlorambucil, nitrogen mustard, busulfan, 5-fluorouracil, or actinomycine D is anagen hair loss. There is cessation of mitosis in the hair bulb, with thinning an constriction of the hair shafts (Pohl-Pinkus constrictions) and breaking at these points. However, these are reversible hair changes, and hair continues to grow. Other drugs that cause alopecia are prolonged, or single high, doses of vitamin A, heparin, coumarin, triparanol, thiourea, carbamazepine, allopurinol, indomethacin, gentamicin, levodopa, propranolol, isotretinoin, entretinate, lithium, and metoprolol.

Stress alopecia after severe and acute emotional upset has been documented. The severe stress of war conditions or acute illness may induce complete hair loss in a matter of a few weeks. It is believed that this is alopecia areata, which may be diffuse, and is identifiable by easy removal of exclamation-point hairs, in children aged one to four or five who have experienced a serious fright.

Congenital alopecia occurs either as total or partial loss of hair, accompanied usually by other ectodermal defects of the nails, teeth, and bone. The hair is light and sparse, and grows slowly. Congenital triangular alopecia and aplasia cutis congenita are examples of congenital localized absence of hair.

SYNDROMES THAT INCLUDE
ABNORMALITIES OF THE HAIR

Polyostotic fibrous dysplasia (Albright's disease) may present — as it did in a case reported by Shelley and Wood - as slowly progressive lifelong unilateral hair loss: scalp, pubic, axillary, and palpebral.

Sickle cel disease is often characterized by scantiness of body and facial hair.

The Cronkhite-Canada syndrome is characterized by alopecia, skin pigmentation, onychodystrophy, malabsorption, and generalized gastro-intestinal polyposis.

Marinesco-Sjogren syndrome consists of cerebellar ataxia, mental retardation, congenital cataracts, inability to chew food, thin brittle fingernails, and sparse hair. The dystrophic hairs do not have the normal layers (cortex, cuticle, and medulla), and 30 percent of the hair shafts show narrow bands of abnormal incomplete keratinization. There is an autosomal recessive type of inheritance in this syndrome.

Trichothiodystrophy features brittle hair with a markedly reduced sulfur content. The hair, with sulfur reduced to 50 percent of the normal value, has distinctive features under polarizing light, and scanning electron microscopy. With polarizing microscopy, the hair shows alternating bright and dark regions which give a striking striped appearance.

In addition to the hair findings, which are present in all cases, other variable features of the syndrome include short stature, mental deficiency, ichthyosis, nail dystrophy, ocular dysplasia, and infertility.

Crow-Fukase ("POEMS") syndrome is characterized by polyneuropathy, organomegaly, endocrinopathy, M-protein, and skin changes such as diffuse hyperpigmentation, dependent edema, skin thickening, hyperhidrosis, and hypertrichosis.

Cartilage-hair hypoplasia consists of short-limbed dwarfism and abnormally fine and sparse hair in children. They are especially susceptible to viral infections and recurrent respiratory infections.

Acquired Immunodeficiency Syndrome Many black patients with AIDS have experienced softening, straightening, lightening, and thinning of their hair.

Tricho-rhino-phalangeal syndrome is a genetic disorder consisting of fine and sparse scalp hair, thin nails, pear-shaped broad nose, and cone-shaped epiphyses of the middle phalanges of some fingers and toes.

Lipidematous alopecia associated with skin hyperelasticity and hyperlaxity of the joints. The alopecia consists of shortened hairs, with thickening of the scalp associated with an increase in subcutaneous fat, so that the scalp may be as much as 15 mm thick.

Hallermann-Streiff syndrome is a rare syndrome of birdlike facies with a pronounced beak-like nose, microphthalmia, micrognathia, congenital cataracts, and hypotrichosis. The hair is diffusely sparse and brittle. Baldness may occur frontally or at the scalp margins, but sultural alopecia, hair loss following the lines of the cranial sutures, is characteristic of this syndrome. The small face is in sharp contrast with a disproportionately large-appearing head. The lips are thin; some of the teeth may be absent while others are dystrophic, resulting in malocclusion. Nystagmus, strabismus, and other ocular abnormalities are present.

Progeria, also known as Hutchinson-Gilford syndrome, is characterized by premature old age. It is marked by failure to develop normally in growth after the first year of life. The large bald head and lack of eyebrows and eyelashes are distinctive. The skin is wrinkled, pigmented, and atrophic. The nails are thin and atrophic. Most patients lack subcutaneous fat, which produces the appearance of premature senility. The intelligence remains intact. Arteriosclerosis, anginal attacks, and hemiplegia may occur, followed by death from coronary heart disease at an early age.

Papillon-Lefevre syndrome is characterized by hyperkeratosis palmaris et plantaris, periodontosis, and sparsity of the hair. Hyperhidrosis and the other signs and symptoms begin early in life. Inheritance of this disease is of an autosomal recessive type.

Klippel-Feil syndrome consists of a low posterior scalp hair line extending onto the shoulders, with a short neck, limiting movement of the neck, and suggestive of webbing. The cervical vertebrae are fused. This syndrome is caused by the faulty segmentation of the mesodermal somites between the third and seventh weeks in utero. Strabismus, nystagmus, cleft palate, bifid uvula, and high palate are some other features. This syndrome occurs mostly in girls.

McCusick's syndrome includes short-limbed dwarfism and fine, sparse, hypoplastic and dysmorphic hair

Turner's syndrome is a distinctive clinical picture comprising short stature, webbing of the neck, low posterior hair line margin, increased carrying angle at the elbow (cubitus valgus), and infantile development of the breasts, vagina, and uterus. Coarctation of the aorta is frequently found. A triangular-shaped mouth, alopecia of the frontal area of the scalp, and cutis laxa are also seen.

Turner's syndrome is caused by ovarian dysgenesis. Only 45 chromosomes are present; the sex chromosomes have an XO pattern.

Noonan's syndrome consists of short stature with typical webbing of the neck, low hair line in the back, prominent and low-set ears, and cubitus valgus.

The syndrome is similar to Turner's syndrome and has been frequently termed "male Turner's syndrome", in which a normal chromosome pattern is assumed.

Werner's syndrome has the essential features of shortness of stature, cataracts, skin changes, premature graying and alopecia, atrophy of muscles and subcutaneous tissues, and bone atrophy of the extremities to produce "spindly extremities". Osteoporosis and aseptic necrosis are frequent in the small bones of the hands.

The skin changes include poikiloderma, scleroderma, atrophy, hyperkeratoses, and leg ulcers. The skin shows a dark gray of blackish diffuse pigmentation. A high-pitched voice and hypogonadism in both sexes are distinctive in this syndrome. Diabetes mellitus is frequently present.

Rothmund-Thomson syndrome is characterized by early-onset poikiloderma, short stature, sun sensitivity, bone defects, and hypogonadism. Cataracts are seen in some families (Rothmund type), and sparseness of eyelashes, eyebrows, or scalp hair has been reported in 60 per cent of cases.

HAIR COLOR

On the basis of the ultrastructure of hair pigment, Mottag and Zelickson have reported the variations in the melanocytes and melano-somes as seen in the different colored hairs. Melanin in the hair follicles is produced in the cytoplasm of the melanocytes, in which are involved the endoplasmic reticulum, ribosomes, and the Golgi apparatus. Melanin synthesis begins on the matrix fibers of the premelanosomes, forming inm the cytoplasm of the melanocytes. Hair color will depend upon the degree of melanin synthesis, on matrix fibers and in the intervening spaces between the fibers. When all tyrosinase activity halts, the premelanosome becomes a melanosome.

The pigment in black and dark brown hair is comoposed of eumelanin, whereas in blond and red hair is a pheomelanin. In

23

black hair the melano-cytes contain the densest melanosomes, with lightened areas that show a "month-eaten" appearance. **Brown hair** differs only by its smaller melanosomes; light brown hair consist of a mixture of the melanosomes of dark hair and the incomplete melanosomes of **blond hair.** Many of the melanosomes in blond hair develop only on the matrix fibers and not in the spaces between the fibers.

Red hair shows incomplete melanin deposits on the matrix fibers to produce a "splotchy" appearing melanosome. Pheomelanin is distinguished by its relatively high content of sulfur, which results from the addition of cysteine to dopaquinone along the biosynthetic pathway of melanin synthesis.

Change in hair color occur in various metabolic disorders. The hair becomes blond in phenylketonuria because of inadequate amounts of tyrosine; in homocystinuria a bleaching effect on the hair is noted; light hair is also seen in oast-house disease; albinism is associated with white or yellowish hair; triparanol is associated with hypopigmented hair; minoxidil (by changing vellus to terminal hairs) causes darkening of hair; another hypotensive agent, diazoxide, gives the hair a reddish tint; in Menkes's kinky hair syndrome the hair is light; in kwashiorkor the hair assumes a red-blond color in infants; with chloroquine therapy depigmentation may occur, usually in redheads and blonds, not in brunettes. Segmental heterochromia, with alternating light and dark bands, may occur in iron deficiency anemia. The disorder has been called canities segmentata sideropenica. It responds completely to iron supplementation.

In **grey hair** (canities) melanogenic activity is decreased as a result of fewer melanocytes and melanosomes as well as a gradual loss of tyrosinase activity. Graying of the scalp hair is genetically determined and may start at any age. Usually it begins at the temples and progresses with time. The beard usually follows, with the body hair coming last.

Early graying (before age 20 in whites or before age 30 in blacks) is usually familial; however, it may occur also in progeria, in the syndromes of Rothmund and Thomson, in Book's syndrome, and in Werner's syndrome.

24

In poliosis, gray hair occurs in circumscribed patches. This may occur in Waardenburg's syndrome and piebaldism and is frequent in tuberous sclerosis. Poliosis is also found in association with vitiligo and Vogt-Koyanagi syndrome and may be seen in alopecia areata when the new hairs grow in. Other syndrome which include poliosis are Tietz's syndrome, Alezzandrini's syndrome, and neurofibromatosis.

Premature whitening of scalp hair is usually due to vitiligo, sometimes with recognized, or actually without, lesions of glabrous skin.

2

HYPERTRICHOSIS

Hypertrichosis is an overgrowth of hair not localized to the androgen dependent areas of the skin. Several forms exist.

Localized Acquired Hypertrichosis. Beighton first reported a curious and rare anomaly, hairy elbows, in 1970. It is a progressive excessive growth of lanugo hairs intially, in which the hairs may reach (as in Andreev's case) a length of 10 cm. Later they become coarser, but regression has been observed during adolescence. Andreev's case had no endocrine abnormality and was not familial. Rudolph, who reported a case in 1985, emphasized the lack of need for endocrine or other studies, since the condition appears to be of only cosmetic significance.

Lupton and Odom have seen two patients with excessive growth of lanugo hairs on the anterior neck just above the suprasternal notch.

Dermal tumors, such as melanocytic nevi or Becker's nevi, may have excessive terminal hair growth. Repeated irritation, trauma, occlusion under a cast, eczematous states, topical steroid use, linear melo-rheostotic scleroderma, the Crow-Fukase (POEMS) syndrome, and pretibial myxedema may be other situations in which there is localized increase in hair growth. Porphyrias generally show a localized hypertrichosis over the malar area such as in porphyria cutanea tarda or variegate prophyria;

Localized Congenital Hypertrichosis. Such cases include congenital nevocytic nevi, simple nevoid hypertrichosis, or as a sign of underlying spinal dysraphism (when occurring over the sacral midline).

Generalized Congenital Hypertrichosis (Congenital Hypertrichosis Lanuginosa). Beighton summarized this rare type of excessive and generalized hairiness, inherited by

27

autosomal dominance. His patient, a boy of five years, was covered over his entire body with fine vellus hairs 2 to 10 cm long. The scalp hair appeared to be normal; otherwise, with the exception of the palms and soles, all areas were covered. Congenital hypertrichosis lanuginosa may be associated with dental anomalies and gingival fibromatosis. This type of hairiness has attracted considerable attention over the centuries. These unfortunately afflicted individuals have been billed as "dog-face boy", "human werewolf," and "human Skye terrier."

Other cases of congenital generalized hypertrichosis may be secondary to drug ingestion by the mother. The fetal hydantoin syndrome is characterized by hypertrichosis, depressed nasal bridge, large lips, a wide mouth, and a short, webbed neck. The fetal alcohol syndrome includes hypertrichosis, a small face, capillary hemangiomas, and physical and mental retardation. A case of generalized hypertrichosis and multiple congenital defects was reported by Kaler et al in a baby born to a mother who used minoxidil throughout pregency.

Generalized or Patterned Acquired Hypertrichosis. These cases include those due to acquired hypertrichosis lanuginosa, those associated with various syndromes, and those secondary to drug intake. Syndromes associated with increased hair growth include lipoatrophic diabetes, Ruben-stein-Tylor syndrome (craniofacial dysostosis and patent ductus arteriosua), Cornelia de Lange's syndrome, Hurler's syndrome, Morogu's syndrome, leprechaunism, Winchester's syndrome, and the Schynzel-Giedier syndrome. Drugs associated with hypertrichosis include minoxidil, cyclosporine, diphenylhydantoin, diazoxide, streptomycine, penicillamine, corticosteroids, danazol, psoralens, hexachlorobenzene, and topical steroids or topical androgens.

3

HIRSUTISM

CLINICAL FEATURES. Hirsutism is an excess of terminal hair growth in women in a pattern more typical of men. Androgen-dependent growth areas affected include the upper lip, cheeks, chin, the central chest, the breasts, and the lower abdomen and groins. This altered growth pattern of the hair may or may not be associated with other signs of virilization, which include temporal balding, masculine habitus, deepening of the voice, clitoral hypertrophy, and amenorrhea. Acne is an additional associated phenomenon in some cases of hirsutism. When virilization accompanies hirsutism, especially when progression is rapid, a neoplastic cause is likely. Neoplastic causes account for only a small minority of hirsute women.

PATHOGENESIS. Racial variation should be considered when evaluating hirsutism. Women of Middle Eastern, Russian, and Southern European countries commonly have facial, abdominal, and thigh hair, whereas Oriental and Indian women generally have little terminal hair growth in these areas.

In women, androgen biosynthesis occurs only in the ardenal and the overy. The potent androgen testosterone and the androgen precursor androstenedione are secreted by the ovary. The adrenal contributions are preandrogens; dehydroepiandrosterone (DHEA), DHEA sulfate, and androstenedione require peripheral conversion in the skin and liver to testosterone.

Testosterone is converted to dihydrotestosterone, the androgen that promotes androgen-dependent hair growth, in the hair follicle by 5 alpha-reductase. Receptor molecules in the end organ are necessary for binding and hormone action at that level. Since testosterone is normally bound to carrier molecules in the plasma at a 99 per cent level, and it is the unbound testosterone which is active, the levels of free testosterone

29

reflect clinical evidence of androgen excess, rather than total testosterone.

Hirsutism, then, may result either from excessive secretion of androgrens from either the ovary of the adrenal gland, or from excessive stimulation by pituitary tumors. The excessive secretion may be from functional excesses or from neoplastic processes. All cases of severe or progressive hirsutism should be investigated for an endocrinopathy.

Ovarian causes include polycystic ovary disease (Stein-Leventhal syndrome), and a variety of ovarian tumors, both benign and malignant. The Stein-Leventhal syndrome is characterized by hirsutism (50 per cent), acne (20 per cent), and signs such as amenorrhea, uterine bleeding, anovulation, obesity, and small breasts. The ovaries are frequently palpable on physical examination, as they are polycystic. Pelvic ultrasound is useful also; however, culdoscopy and colpotomy may be necessary for diagnosis. Serum free testosterone is generally elevated. Luteinizing hormone is also elevated, but follicle-stimulating hormone levels remain normal or may be decreased. Ovarian tumors include unilateral benign microadenomas, arrhenoblastomas, Leydig cell tumors, hilarcell tumors, granular-thecal cell tumors, and luteomas. Here the onset is usually rapid, occurs with associated virilization, and begins between the ages of 20 and 40. Again free testosterone is high (generally greater than 2 ng/ml).

Adrenal causes include congenital adrenal hyperplasia and adrenal tumors such as adrenal adenomas and carcinomas. The adrenogenital syndrome or congenital adrenal hyperplasia is an autosomal dominant disorder which may result from deficiencies of the following enzymes: 21-hydroxylase (most common form), 11-hydroxylase, and 3b-hydroxy steroid dehydrogenase. Onset is generally in childhood, with ambiguous genitalia, precocious growth, and virilism; however, adult-onset types with partial enzyme deficiencies present generally with hirsutism as a familial trait.

Pituitary causes include Cushing's disease, acromegaly, and prolactin-secreting adenomas. Cushing's disease and acromegaly are dealt with in Chapter 24. Prolactin-secreting microadenomas have a 20 per cent incidence of hirsutism and acne. Other conditions in which prolactin levels may be elevated and which may lead to hirsutism include hypothyroidism, phenothiazine intake, and hepato-renal failure.

Other causes of hirsutism include the exogenous intake of androgens and certain high-progesterone birth control pills (uncommonly). End-organ hypersensitivity may be a mechanism in patients with a normal evaluation. Drugs such as minoxidil, diazoxide, corticosteroids, and phenytoin, which have been reported as causing hirsutism, generally cause hypertrichosis — a generalized increase in hair not limited to the androgen-sensitive areas.

EVALUATION. A careful history and physical examination are essential. The history should focus on onset and progression, virilization, menstrual history, and family/racial background. Physical examination may reveal signs of Cushing's disease or acromegaly. Other signs to be evaluated are the distribution of muscle mass and body fat, clitoral dimensions, voice depth, and galactorrhea.

Laboratory evaluation should include a free testosterone level, a dehydroepiandrosterone sulfate level, a 17-hydroxy progesterone level, and a prolactin level.

TREATMENT. Once appropriate testing has led to diagnosis and referral of patients requiring special methods of specific treatment, such as surgical intervention, therapeutic alternatives include cosmetic (mechanical) treatments, nonspecific suppressive therapy, and specific antiandrogens.

Cosmetic or mechanical methods of treatment are the cheapest and easiest methods, and expose the patient to the fewest potential side effects. Shaving is best; however, it is often the most resisted, due to social influences. Wax depilatories, chemical depilatories, bleaching of the hair, and electrolysis are alternatives.

Epilating waxes, usually made of beeswax and rosin, are satisfactory for temporary removal of moderate amounts of cosmetically objectionable hair. It has been proved beyond a doubt that the temporary removal of hairs by waxes, shaving ,

31

or plucking does not stimulate their growth or coarsen subsequent growth.

Depilatories containing barium sulfide corrode the projecting hair shaft, but have no destructive action on the intrafollicular growing portion. The barium sulfide may irritate the skin excessively, making this procedure undesirable.

Bleaching with hydrogen peroxide with or without equal parts of strong ammonia makes dark hairs less noticeable and corrodes the finer hairs. Before it is applied, the skin is cleaned with ether to remove any oiliness. It is advisable to begin with one tenth of the usual strength.

Epilation with the use of a high frequency or galvanic current is a safe method for the permanent removal of superfluous hair. A certain number of recurrences (20 to 35 per cent) is inevitable even when it is done by experts. Such hairs must be removed a second time. Referral to an "electrologist" is suggested.

Attempts to cure hypertrichosis by x-rays are about as old as x-rays. Permanent epilation can be effected by x-rays only when sufficient exposure is given to cause subsequent permanent damage to the skin. Numerous sad cases of radiodermatitis, skin keratoses, and cancers have been produced by x-rays used for epilation. It should never be done.

These mechanical modalities should be used at least initially, even when medical treatment is planned. In order to achieve some early response, since medical intervention takes many months to give a noticeable response.

Nonspecific suppressive therapies include oral contraceptives and glucocorticoids. Practically, these therapies suppress hirsutism due to adrenal or overian causes equally, and hence are utilized based on the individual patient's wants and needs, with particular attention to the specific effects of medication.

4

CARE OF THE HAIR

It consists of:—

Washing with soap or shampoo. Sometimes beaten egg white is employed to give glossiness to the hair. Sunny, Weleda Calendula are useful in controlling dandruff. In India, certain indigenous plant products like ritha and amla are used for washing the hair. They are cheap and effective. Greasy hair need frequent washing and less oil application. Dry hair require less frequent washing and good oil massage. Frequency of washing depends upon the climate and the length of the hair, daily, alternate days or weekly. Often bland soap and water are sufficient.

Greasing or oil application is essential for effective lubrication and grooming; choice depends upon individual taste.

Combing and brushing of the hair is normally done once or twice a day. No force should be used in either combing or brushing. Combs and brushes tend to irritate the scalp; often injures and atrophies the hair.

Singeing of the hair ends is often employed by beauty palours and hairdressers to treat splitting. It has no advantages over cutting, and is by no means curative.

Dyeing grey hair with vegetable dyes (henna, chamomile), metallic dyes (bismuth, silver, lead) and chemical dyes (paratolyendiamine, paraphenylnediamine, etc.). Several dye preparations are available in the market. Vegetable dyes are usually the safest, but there is limited choice of colour in them. Patch test to the dye must be applied before its use.

Permanent waving, and straightening of wooly hair (as in Negroes).

Broadly speaking there are two methods of permanent waving:—

a) *The cold method:* The hair is curled by means of curlers and softened with a reducing agent like ammonium thioglycolate so that it can conform to the undulations made by the curlers; later, undulations are fixed with a neutralizer or an oxidising agent.

b) *The hot method:* The hair is first softened by an alkaline sulphate solution, and then undulations are made by rods and the application of heat (electrical, steam or chemicals).

The hair is shampooed before any of the two techniques of permanent waving are employed. Burning of the scalp by direct heat, or chemical irritation and sensitization are some of the risks of permanent waving. Due precautions should be taken; patch tests should precede the use of chemicals

Hair ornaments: Pins, clips and nets. These are employed to keep the hair in a desired shape and also to enhance looks. Only rarely do such accessories cause dermatitis. Nickel and plastic materials should be used with caution to prevent irritation. Wigs are worn, particularly by women, to conceal alopecia or for improving appearance.

5

Therapeutics of Hair Loss

Acid fluor: Itching of the head and falling of the hair after fevers; the new hair is dry and breaks off; must comb the hair often. It mats so at the end.

Aloes: The hair come out in lumps, leaving bare patches; eyelashes also fall out; dry hair;

Aluminia: Hair fall from all over body including lashes. Denuded appearance of scalp. Itching and numbness of scalp. Dandruff.

Ammonium mur: Large accumulation of branlike scales, with falling off of the hair, which has a deadened and lustreless of appearance, with great itching of the scalp.

Anantherum: Falling of hair from beard and eyebrows.

Antimonium crud: Losing hair from nervous headaches. Itching of the head.

Arsenicum: Touching the hair is painful; bald patches at or near the forehead, bregma, sides, scalp covered with dry scabs and scales, looking rough and dirty extending sometimes even to forehead, face and ears. Brittle and stiff hair. Dandruff.

Aurum: Syphilitic alopecia.

Baryta carb: Hairfall from vertex and moustache. Baldness, especially of the crown, in young people; scalp very senstive to touch < from scratching, touch.

Belladona: Hair fall from eyebrows and bregma brittle hair.

Borax: Hair rough & horny. Tangles at tips, sticks

35

together. If bunches are cut they reform. Hair can't be combed smooth - especially occiput, sides, vertex, temples, beard, nostrils.

Bovista: Hair fall from sides.

Calcarea carb: Hair falls out, especially when combing; dryness of hair; great sensitiveness of scalp, with yellowish or white scales on scalp; sensation of coldness of outer head.

Calcarea Phos: Falling of hair in bunches.

Cantharis: Hair falls out in bunches, spots when combing, especially during confinement and lactation; scales on scalp, enormous dandruff, stiff hair.

Carbo veg.: Falling out of hair after severe diseases or abuse of mercury, with great sensitiveness of scalp to pressure; hair falls out more on back of head, after severe illness or parturition. Hair fall worse from warmth of head, cold sweat on forehead.

Causticum: Hair fall from eyebrows and nostrils.

China: Hair sweats much (Bry) and falls out. Sore, sensitive

Scalp < touching

< combing.

Colchicum: Prurigo favosa; great falling of the hair.

Fluoric acid: Hair fall after syphilis,, fevers. Large patches entirely denuded of hair; new hair brittle, dry and breaks off; must comb the hair often; it mats so at the end; baldness. Hair in tangles, congestion of blood to the head.

Graphites: Even the hair on the sides of the head, vertex and nostrils falls out. Dry, tangled, matted or brittle hair. Perspiration of scalp, greying of hair. Dandruff, like milk crusts.

Helleborus:	Losing hair from the eyebrows or pudenda.
Hepar:	Hair fall after parturition. Hair falls out here and there - vertex, occiput, bregma leaving bald spots. Scalp sore and senstive.
Hypericum:	Alopecia from headaches, caused by concussion of the brain.
Iodum:	Falling of hair after injury. Hair fall in bunches — stiff hair.
Kali Carb:	Alopecia after nervous fevers; dry brittle hair, rapidly falling off from eyebrow, temple, beard, moustache and sides with much dandruff. Greying of hair.
Lechesis:	Hairfall especial in pregency. Sensitive scalp. Does not want hair touched.
Lycopodium:	Hair fall from temples and vertex. Hair becomes grey early; hair falls off after abdominal diseases; after parturition, with burning, scalding, itching of the scalp, especially on getting warm from exercise during the day. Dandruff.
Mancinella:	Losing hair after severe acute diseases.
Mercurius:	Hair falls out mostly on sides and eyelashes, bregma, temples, without any headache. Greasy hair.
Mezercum:	Hairfall in handfuls. Curly hair. Hair sticks together. Thick leathery crusts under which pus collects. White scabs and dandruff.
Natrum mur:	Hair fall after nursing. Hair falls out if touched: mostly on forepart of head, bregma, moustache, temples and beard; scalp very sensitive; face shining as if greasy. Dandruff on occiput.
Nitric acid:	Hair fall from beard and vertex.
Petroleum:	Much itching; scurf on the hairy scalp and

falling off of the hair in bunches, spots especially from occiput.

Phosphoric acid: Hair fall after grief, anguish and debility especially from sides. Gnawing grief changes hair of the young to grey; Dry, greasy and fluffy hair. Hairfall from the sides.

Phosphorus: Hair fall after mental emotion or sickness. Round patches on scalp completely deprived of hair; falling off the hair in large bunches on the tufts, occiput, forehead and on the sides above the ears; the roots of the hair seems to be dry; the denuded scalp looks clear white and smooth; dandruff copious, falls out in clouds. Itching of the scalp.

Plumbum: Great dryness of hair, it falls off even in beard.

Sabina: Hair fall from temples.

Sarsaparilla: Mercurio-syphilitic affections of the head; sensitiveness of scalp; falling of the hair.

Selenium: Hair falls off when combing; also of eyebrows, whiskers, vertex, eyelaches and genitals; tingling, itching on scalp, which feels tense and contracted. Does not want hair touched.

Sepia: Hair fall after chronic headaches and menopause especially from vertex and occiput, worse when combing. Itching of root of hair.

Silicea: Premature baldness, itching of scalp or of vulva before menses. Hair fall from vertex, occiput, bregma beard and nostrils after headaches or perturition.

Staphisagria: Hair falls out, mostly from occiput, eylashes, sides and around the ears, with humid, foetid eruption or dandruff on the scalp. Hair pulls out without pain after the slightest effort; offensiveness. Head lice.

Sulphur:	Hair fall after parturition. Hair fall from occiput and eyelashes. Dandruff, hair dry, falling off, scalp sore to touch, itching violently < when getting warm in bed and washing. Hair grey, offensive, dry, cold and hard.
Syphilinum:	Hair falls out after syphilis, in circles from heard and scalp.
Thallium:	Hair fall after excessive perspiration of scalp and after acute exhausting diseases.
Thuja:	White, scaly dandruff; hair dry and falling out. Hairfall after headache, from vertex. Dry or greasy hair, lusterless and split. Gray hair.
Thyroidinum:	Premature graying of hair.
Vinca minor:	Hair falls out in single spots and white hair grows there; spots on head oozing moisture, the hair matting together. Bald patches covered. Itching of scalp with short wooly hair.
Wiesbaden:	Hairfalls and grows rapidly. Hard, brittle and lustreless hair.
Zincum:	Hair fall from sides and vertex.

6

HAIR

FALLING
Alum, *Ambr*, Amm-C, *Amm-m*, *Ant-c*, Ant-t, Apis, Arn, *Ars*, Ars-iod, *Arund*, Asc-t, *Aur*, *Aur-m*, Aur-m-n, Aur-s, *Bar-c*, Bell, *Bor*, Boc, Boy, Bry, Bufo, *Calc-c*, *Calc-p*, Calc-S, *Canth*, *Carb-an*, **Carb-s, Carb-veg.**, Carl, Caust, *Chel*, Chlol, Chin, Colch, *Con*, Cop, *Dulc*, Elaps, *Ferr*, Ferr-ars, Ferr-m, Ferr-p, **Flu-ac**, *Form*, Glon, **Graph**, Hell, *Hepar*, *Ign*, Iod, Kali-ars, *Kali-bi*, **Kali-c**, Kali-iod, Kali-nit, Kali-p, **Kali-S**, Kreos, **Lach, Hyco**, *Mag-c*, Manc, *Merc*, *Merc-cor*, *Mez*, Naja, Nat-c, **Nat-m**, Nat-p **Nit-ac**, Nuph, Oena, Op, Osm, *Par*, *Petr*, *Phosp-ac*, **Phosp**, Plb Psor, *Rhust*, Rhus-v, Sab, San, Sars, Sec, *Sel*, **Sepia, Silicea**, *Staph*, **Sulph**, Sulph-ac, Syph, Tab, Tep, **Thuj**, Thyr, Tub, Ust, Vesp, *Zinc*.

SPOTS:—ALOPECIA AREATA
Alum, *Apis*, *Ars*, *Calc-c*, Calc-p, Canth, Carb-an, **Flu-ac**, *Hep*, **Iod**, *Lyco*, *Nat-m*, Petr, *Phosp, Psor*

BEARD:
Agar, Ambr, Anan, Aur-m, *Calc-c*, Carb-an, *Graph*, *Kali-c*, *Nat-c*, *Nat-m*, Nit-ac, *Phosp-ac*, Plb, Sanic, Sel, Sil.

BREGMA: (FOREHEAD).
Ars, *Bell*, *Hep-s*, **Merc**, **Nat-m**. **Phosp**, Sil.

EARS: above and behind:- *Phosp.*

EYE BROWS:
Agar, Nil, Alum, *Anan*, Aur-m, **Bell**, *Caust*, Hell, **Kali-c**, Mill, *Par*, Plb, **Sele**, Sil, Sulph.

EYE LASHES:
Alum, *Apis*, *Ars*, Aur, Bor, Bufo, *Calc-s*, *Chel*, Chlol, *Euph*, *Graph*, Med, *Merc*, Nat-m, Phosp-ac, Psor, **Rhus-t**, *Sele*, Sep, Sil, *Staph*, *Sulph*.

MOUSTACHE:
Bar-c, **Kali-c**, **Nat-m**, Plb, Sel.

NOSTRILS:
Calc-c, *Caust*, *Graph*, Iod, Sil.

OCCIPUT:
Calc-c, **Carb-veg**, *Chel*, Hep, Merc, *Petr*, *Phosp*, Sep., Sil,
Staph, Suph.

SIDES:
Ars, Bov., **Calc-C**, *Graph*, Kali-c, Merc. Phosp, Phosp-ac, *Staph*,
Zinc.

TEMPLES:
Calc-c, *Kali-c*, Lyco, Merc, *Nat-m*, Par, Sab.

VERTEX (CROWN)
Alum, *Anac*, *Apis*, Aurum, **Bar-c**, *Calc-c*, Carb-an, *Flu-ac*,
Graph, Hep, Lyco, *Nit-ac*, *Phosp*, Plb, *Sel*, *Sil*, Syph, Thuja,
Zinc.

ROOTS:
destroyed by auption (tinea) - Ars
turn dry and hair gray - Phos
Painful — Arund, Calc, Coloc
Painful on combing — Nat-s
Painful when combed as from ulceration — *Chel*
Pain when hair is moved — CINCH
Painful after scratching — Caps
Painful esp to touch — Cinnab, Sulph
Abdomnal diseases after — LYCO
Bunches in — PHOSP
Children in — *Arund*

CLIMAXIS AT:
Sep.

FEVERS AFTER:
Flu-ac.
tyohoid fever — FLU-AC

42

GRIEF FROM: (Sorrow from)
Phosp-ac
Handfuls in when combing — *Sulph*

HEADACHE AFTER:
Ant-c, Hep-s, Nit-ac, **Sepia**, Sil, Thuja.

HYSTERIA WITH:
Lyco

ILLNESS SEVERE AFTER:
Carb-v, Manc, Thal.

INJURY FROM:
Hyper

LACTATION DURING:
Nat-m.

PARTURITION AFTER:
Calc-c, Canth, Carb-veg, Hep, LYCO. Nat-m, *Nit-ac, Sep,*
Sil, **Sulph.**

PREGENCY DURING:
LACH

TYPE OF HAIR:
Bristling:
Acet-ac, *Acon*, Amm-c, Arn., Bar-c, Calc-c, Canth, Carl, Carb-
veg, *Cham, Chel,* Cina, Cocc-a, Dulc, Lachn, *Haur,* Lyco, Mag-
m, Mang, Meny, Merc., *Mur-ac,* Nit-ac, Nux-v, Puls. Seneg, Sil.
Spong, Sulph-iod, Tarent, Verat. *Zinc.*

Brittle:
Ars, Bell, Flu-ac, Graph, *Kali-c,* Psor.

Bunching of: (Sticking, Tangles, Matted)
Ant-t, *Borax, Flu-ac,* Graph, *Lyco,* **Mez,** *Nat-m, psor,* **Sars,**
Verat, **Vinc.**

Cold:
Sabad.

Constant attempt to tear
in children — Bell
with unconsciousness — Tub
uterine dementia — *Lil-tig*
in peureral convulsions — Ign

Dry:
Aloe, Alum, *Ambr*, Bad, *Calc-c*, Chel, *Flu-ac*, *Graph*, Hipp, *Kali-c*, *Med*, *Phosp*, Phosp-ac, *Plb*, *Psor*, Sec., *Sulph*, **Thuj**.

Fluffy:
Med, Phosp-ac.

Frowsy:
Bor

Gray:
Ars, Graph, Hipp, *Kali-iod*, Kali-nit, Kreos, **Lyc**, Op. *Phosp-ac*,
Sec, *Sil*, Staph, *Sulph*, Sulph-ac, Thuj.

Greasy: (Oily)
Bry, Lac-c, Lyss, **Phosp-ac**, Plb, Thuja,

Growth, slow, short — Thuja

Lustreless:
Flu-ac, **Hippo**, Kali-nit, *Med*, **Psor**, *Thuja*, Tub.
in seborrhoea sicca — Hydras

Offensive:
Bufo, *Lyco*, Staph, Sulph, *Vinca*, Vio-t.

Pulled as if — Aethusa, Caps
headache with — Alum
hemicrania — *Phosp*
as if drawn upward with vertigo — Mur-ac

Stiff:
Ars., Canth, Iod.

Thin — Thuja
in eczema of scalp — Kali.bi
with uterine neuralgia — *Nux-v*

Withered look:
Phosp-ac.

Dandruff:
All-s, Alum, *Amm-m*, *Ars*, Bad, *Bry*, *Calc-c*, *Calc-s*, **Canth**, **Carb-s**, *Dulc*, **Graph**, Kali-c, Kali-chl, Kali-p, *Mali-s*, Lac-c, *Lyco*, Mag-c, *Med*, *Mez*, **Nat-m**, *Olnd*, **Phosp**, *Psor*, Sanic, *Sep*, Stann, *Staph*, **Sulph**, Thuja.

Itching:
Med.

Scaly, (Profuse)
Sanic

White:
Ars, *Kali-chl*, Kali-m. *Mez*, **Nat-m**, *Phosp*, **Thuja**.

Yellow:
Calc-c, **Kali-s**.

7

CASES
CLINICAL CASES OF HAIR FALL

Miss M.T.: has complained of hair falling with flanking of skin of scalp.
Change of colour from black ——> brown
Head pain W Sun
Desires sweets
Desires sour.
Perspiration profuse in axilla.
Moody ——> before menses
Hot patient
Angry when dominated
Impatient
Sensitive

On the following symptoms *Natrum-mur* was selected in 200 potency on 1-6-90. As the response to the medicine was good and the hairfall was showing improvement. *Nat-mur* was given with increasing potencies uptl 10 M then 50 M till 4th June 1991. The patient is showing improvement in the hair fall and also the complaint of headache is better with the medicine.

Miss R.D.: had come with the complaint of hairfall associated with dandruff causing severe itching of the scalp. She also complained of dark circles around the eyes and cracks of the heels.
Myopia
Desires - Spicy food
Desires - meat
Perspiration - axilla
Hot patient
Nervous patient
Obstinate
Confidence lack of
Contradiction < 's
Reserved

Based on the following data, repertorization of the case was done and the remedy *Natrum-mur* was selected, Initially it was given in 30 potency and then gradually increased to 200-1m-10m.

Mrs. T.S.: Complaint of hairfall with dandruff. scaling of scalp, itching in scalp +

                                     < night
                                       < perspiration during
                                       > scratching

         Head pain - throbbing < coughing
                                 < laughing

         Obese person
         Menses irregular
         Leucorrhoea - Before menses
         Perspiration - forehead
         Desires - sour and pungent food.
         Hot patient
         Fear of being alone
         Slowness
         Offended easily
         Sympathetic.

Based on the above symptomatology and after repertorizartion *Phosphorous* was selected in 200 potency later increased to 1M-10,-50M.

Miss S.D.S.: age 6 years came with problem of hairfall with recurrent tendency to catch cold.
         Desires - pickless
         Desires - cold drinks
         Perspiration - forehead
         Fear of dark
         Fear of ghost.
         Restlessness - children in
         Sensitive to reprimands
         Nail biting
After repertorization, *phosphorous* was selected in 30 potency then 200 - 1M - 10M - 50M.

8

HAIR LOSS

Some common questions with their relevant answers regarding hair loss.

Q.1.   What makes hair loss worse?

Whatever the main reasons for hair loss, there are other factors which can make the problems worse, These are:-
a) Rubbing or pulling hair;
b) Stress — when severe or sudden;
c) Serious illness, a high fever or a big operation.
d) Thyroid disease;
e) Anaemia;
f) Following child birth (usually noticed 3 months later).
g) Skin diseases affecting the scalp (e.g. severe dermatitis).
h) Some medicines, especially those used to treat cancer.

Q.2.   Can I myself prevent further hair loss?

If the tendency to lose hair runs in your family, there is nothing you can do to stop it happening to you. But it makes sense to take extra care of your hair, to try and keep the loss down as much as possible.
a)   Be cautious with hair dyes. Don't overuse them, they tend to dry hair and can weaken it.
b)   Vigorous rubbing, scrating or massaging of the scalp can damage hair.
c)   Use a soft-bristled brush-be gentle, don't tug at your hair.
d)   Don't be afraid to use shampoo or hairspray or to have your hair permed.
None of these should cause hair loss.

Q.3.   How can I cope with losing my hair ?

Hair loss can be very distressing especially for women and young men.

It is seen as unglamorous and sign of aging, especially because we are constantly under the misconception that an "ideal body" always has a "full head of hair".

Hair loss is not uncommon and it will not alter the real your or change the way that friends and family feel about you.

If you would like more advice and help, see your Homeopathic physician who will help you about your hair loss for whatever reason.

Q.4.   What can I do to help my remaining hair ?

1) *Hair thickeners* : which coat the hair and give it more body.
2) Women can try a *gentle perm* to lift the hair and make it look fuller.
3) Wearing a *hairpiece* or wig won't harm your remaining hair, but bear in mind that once you've started to wear one regularly, people will notice if you stop. If you decide on a wig, have it thinned out by a hair dresser for a more natural look

Q.5.   How to take care of my hair ?

To make the very best of your hair, you need to look after it with care.

Here are some tips.

Washing :
Scales and grease are produced by the scalp, so they need washing.

How quickly your hair becomes dirty depends on your work and where you live.

Generally, most people need to wash their hair twice a week. Hair can be washed with soap but expect difficulties rinsing it out completely.

It is better to use shampoo which usually contains a detergent, soap, water and oils. Find a mild shampoo which suits your hair. Hair conditioners are important as they reduce the friction between hairs and help to give it body.

Dry :
Do not rub hair roughly with a towel to dry it. Instead pat-dry to remove most of the water and then comb it into place. There is no reason why you should not blow-dry but a lower heat will help to keep your hair healthy. Avoid strong heat because this cracks the hair cuticle making it more likely to split.

Greasy hair :
Greasy hair is a problem for many people, especially when it sticks hairs together to make an already thinning scalp look even balder.

There are special shampoos (containing detergents) which often help, but occasionally may be too strong and make the problem worse. Avoid anti-dandruff shampoos and brushing, and combing your hair a lot, all of which stimulate grease glands.

Dry hair :
Dry hair is due to the scalp not producing as much grease as it should. It may also make an already thinning scalp look balder. Special shampoos which leave more oil behind and contain conditioner to make hair look shiny may help this problem.

Q.6.   What about trichology ?

Trichologists are hair care advisers.

They are mainly helpful for advice about the condition of your hair.

Treatment for hair loss:
Although many treatments have been used to reverse hair loss, there are very few that genuinely make any difference.

Hormones:
Hormones can be used for hair loss to overcome or oppose the effect of male hormones. They cannot be given to men because

51

they cause loss of sex drive and development of female characteristics.

Though some young women are helped, they should not take these hormones for a long time.

Hair Restorants:
Some modern medicines are now being tested as hair restorants.

Success rate of such preparations may be 10-30%. Many products which claim to grow hair are not only inactive but may contain mixtures of chemicals which may harm the hair of scalp.

Hair Transplant:
This is an operation is which strong hairs are taken from the back of the head where it may be growing well and replaced in little groups on the bald places. The disadvantage is that the transplant doesn't always 'take' so the hair may start falling out shortly afterwards. The other problem is that, as time passes, these hairs will also start to thin out just like the hair which originally grew in that area.

Scalp Expansions:
The purpose of this painfull and lengthy process is to expand the skin on the scalp so that the bald areas can be out.

The scalp is stretched with balloons which are placed under the skin and gradually filled with injections. When there is enough spare skin, the bald area is cut out and the edges joined together. It doesn't result in there being any more hairs on the head but they are now spread out over the whole head. Unfortunately they too, continue to thin.

HOMOEOPATHIC TREATMENT FOR LOSS OF HAIR:

Homoeopathic treatment for the loss of hair will be one of the most ideal treatment to be taken from your Homoeopathic physician. Homoeopathic treatment will comprise of complete and detailed case taking by the physician.

After Repertorisation the patients Constitutional medicine is decided taking into consideration the complete totality of the case.

The constitutional medicine will help the patient.
Drugs: for hair falling have been explained later in the book.

9

SOME WORDS EXPLAINED

Androgens:
Male hormones mostly made in the testes. The main one is testosterone. They affect hair growth, often very differently for each part of the body. so, it is possible to have new strong hair growing on the chest or back while starting to lose it from the scalp.

Their balding effect can be overcome in some women by giving female hormones. But this is not possible in men because they would lose sex drive and develop female characteristics.

Alopecia:
The medical word for baldness. There are usually two types.

Common baldness, and alopecia areata in which round, bald patches develop.

Conditioner:
Conditioners improve the look of hair by coating the outside of hairs like varnish on wood and giving them a glossy look. They do not make hair grow more healthy or faster.

Dermis:
Layer of the skin which lies below the epidermis. It is full of a fibrous protein called collagen to make the skin elastic and strong and blood vessels to nourish the skin and take away waste products.

It also has nerve endings, hair follicles, oil flands and sweat glands.

Dermatologists:
Hospital doctor specialising in the care of illness related to the skin, hair and nails.

Epidermis:
Outer layer of the skin. It contains cells to protect structures below, water to keep the skin supple a water proof material hyalin and colour pigment cells.

Follicile:
The lowest part of a hair (root). It lies deeply in the dermis at an angle. It contains cells which divide to form the hair itself.

Hormone:
Chemical substance (like endiogens) produced by a gland (like testes) which is carried in the blood to parts of the body (like the skin) where it has an effect.

Lanugo:
A layer of fine hairs which covers an unborn baby. It is often still there at birth but disappears soon afterwards.

Melanin:
Colour pigment found on the skin shaft of hair and eyes. It absorbs the dangerous ultra violet light produced by the sun. So those with fair skin (little pigment) are more at risk of skin cancers than those with dark pigment (a lot of pigment)

Steroids:
Chemicals with many functions which circulate round the body. One function is to reduce inflammation and allergy which is why it sometimes successfully treats alopecia areata.

Shampoo:
Shampoo contains detergents, water and oils. There are different types for greasy, dry and normal hair. Most people need about two washes a week, applying shampoo once each wash.

Trichologist:
Hair care adviser.

Vellus:
Fine hair which grows everywhere except on palms and soles and anywhere coarse hair grows.

10

Bibliograpic References

Andrews diseases of the skin — 8th Edition 1990.

Colour Atlas of Dermatology — 3rd edition 1986

Practice of Dermatology (P.N. Behl) — 6th edition 1987

Synthetic Repertory (Barthel and Klunker) — 3rd edition 1990

Repertory of the Homoeopathic Materia Medica (J T Kent) — 6th edition 1990

A course repertory of Homoeopathic Medicines (Dr. S.R. Phatak) — 2nd edition 1985

Boericke's Materia Medica with repertory (William Boericke) — 9th edition 1991

Kent's Repertorium Generale (Jost Kunzte) — 1st edition 1987

Repertory of Hering's guiding Symptoms of our Materia Medica (Calvin B. Kuerr) — 1st edition 1986

Boenninghauesen's Characteristics and Repertory (C.M. Boger) — 3rd edition

Homoeopathic Vade Mecum (E Harris Ruddock)

Diseases of the skin (F.M. Dearborn)

Dictionary of Materia Medica (J.H. Clerke)

Homoeopathic Therapeutics (S Lilienthel)

Practical Homoeopathic Therapeutics (W.A. Dewey)

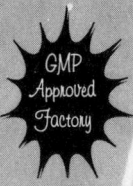
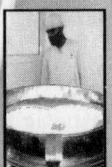
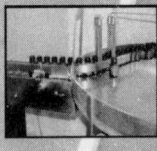
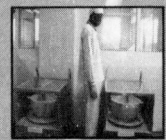
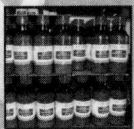
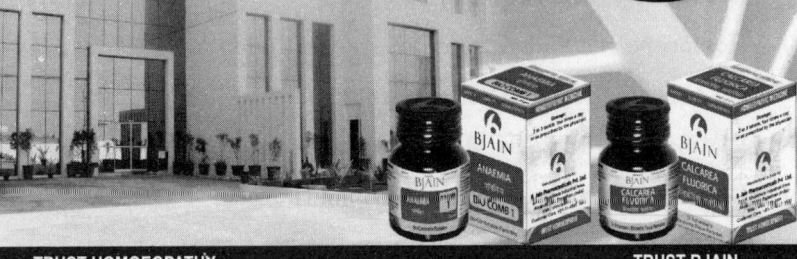